TYPE 2 DIABETES COOKBOOK FOR SENIORS

Manage Type 2 Diabetes with a 30-Day Meal Plan for Seniors

T. John

COPYRIGHT PAGE

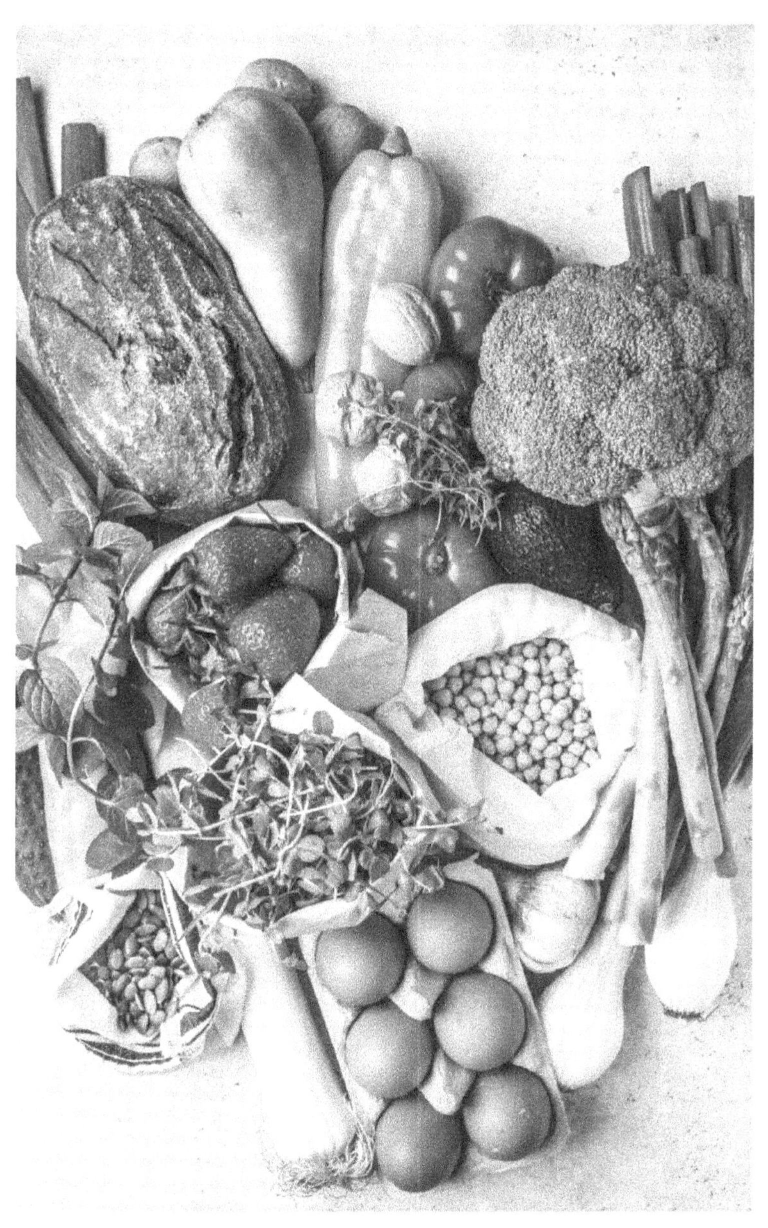

TABLE OF CONTENTS

Chapter 5: Snacks and Appetizers 83

INTRODUCTION

As our bodies age, so too do our metabolic processes. For seniors, this often means an increased risk of developing type 2 diabetes, a chronic condition that affects the body's ability to process sugar. While the diagnosis can be daunting, it's important to remember that with proper management, seniors can live long and fulfilling lives.

Understanding Type 2 Diabetes:

Type 2 diabetes occurs when the body either doesn't produce enough insulin, the hormone responsible for regulating blood sugar, or becomes resistant to its effects. This results in elevated blood sugar levels, which can lead to a host of complications such as heart disease, stroke, nerve damage, and vision problems.

The Significance of Healthy Eating:

For seniors with type 2 diabetes, healthy eating becomes one of the most powerful tools for managing blood sugar levels.

A well-balanced diet rich in fruits, vegetables, whole grains, and lean protein provides essential nutrients while minimizing spikes in blood sugar. Additionally, limiting processed foods, sugary drinks, and unhealthy fats plays a crucial role in maintaining good health.

Essential Dietary Tips for Seniors:

1. **Focus on Whole Foods**: Prioritize whole grains, fruits, and vegetables over refined carbohydrates. Opt for brown rice over white, and choose colorful vegetables like broccoli, carrots, and spinach.

2. **Choose Lean Protein**: Lean protein sources like fish, chicken, beans, and lentils are essential for building and maintaining muscle mass.

3. **Limit Unhealthy Fats**: Reduce your intake of saturated and trans fats found in processed foods, fried foods, and fatty meats. Opt for healthy fats like olive oil, avocado, and nuts.

4. **Mind Your Portions**: Pay attention to portion sizes, as overeating can lead to blood sugar spikes. Use

smaller plates, measure your portions, and avoid
sugary snacks between meals.

5. **Stay Hydrated**: Drinking plenty of water throughout
the day helps regulate blood sugar levels and
promotes overall health.

Managing Blood Sugar Levels:

In addition to healthy eating, managing blood sugar levels
often involves other strategies:

1. **Regular Exercise**: Engaging in regular physical
activity, even if it's just brisk walking, can
significantly improve blood sugar control. Aim for at
least 30 minutes of moderate-intensity exercise most
days of the week.

2. **Monitoring Blood Sugar**: Regularly checking your
blood sugar levels allows you to track your progress
and make necessary adjustments to your diet and
medication.

3. **Medication**: For some seniors, medication may be
necessary to manage blood sugar effectively. Consult

your doctor to determine the best treatment plan for you.

4. **Support System**: Building a strong support system, whether it's family, friends, or a diabetes support group, can provide invaluable emotional and practical assistance.

Remember, age is just a number: By taking control of their health through healthy eating, regular exercise, and proper medication, seniors with type 2 diabetes can lead active and fulfilling lives well into their golden years.

Chapter 1: 30-Day Meal Plan

Week 1:

Day 1:

- Breakfast: Quinoa Breakfast Bowl
- Lunch: Grilled Chicken Salad with Vinaigrette
- Dinner: Baked Cod with Lemon and Herbs
- Snack: Hummus and Veggie Sticks
- Dessert: Sugar-Free Blueberry Muffins

Day 2:

- Breakfast: Veggie Omelette with Whole Grain Toast
- Lunch: Lentil and Vegetable Soup
- Dinner: Sweet Potato and Chickpea Curry
- Snack: Greek Yogurt Dip with Cucumber Slices
- Dessert: Dark Chocolate-Dipped Strawberries

Day 3:

- Breakfast: Greek Yogurt Parfait with Berries
- Lunch: Turkey and Avocado Wrap
- Dinner: Grilled Vegetable and Chicken Kebabs

- Snack: Baked Kale Chips
- Dessert: Baked Apples with Cinnamon

Day 4:

- Breakfast: Spinach and Feta Breakfast Wrap
- Lunch: Quinoa and Black Bean Bowl
- Dinner: Spinach and Mushroom Stuffed Pork Tenderloin
- Snack: Apple Slices with Almond Butter
- Dessert: Berry and Yogurt Popsicles

Day 5:

- Breakfast: Chia Seed Pudding with Almond Milk
- Lunch: Salmon and Asparagus Foil Pack
- Dinner: Beef and Broccoli Stir-Fry
- Snack: Guacamole with Whole Grain Pita Chips
- Dessert: Almond Flour Chocolate Chip Cookies

Day 6:

- Breakfast: Whole Grain Pancakes with Sugar-Free Syrup
- Lunch: Chickpea and Spinach Stew

- Dinner: Cauliflower Crust Pizza with Vegetables
- Snack: Cottage Cheese with Pineapple Chunks
- Dessert: Greek Yogurt and Berry Parfait

Day 7:

- Breakfast: Avocado and Tomato Breakfast Sandwich
- Lunch: Tuna Salad Lettuce Wraps
- Dinner: Quinoa-Stuffed Acorn Squash
- Snack: Mixed Nuts and Seeds Trail Mix
- Dessert: Avocado Chocolate Mousse

Week 2:

Day 8:

- Breakfast: Berry and Spinach Smoothie Bowl
- Lunch: Cauliflower Fried Rice with Shrimp
- Dinner: Shrimp and Vegetable Skewers
- Snack: Edamame with Sea Salt
- Dessert: Pumpkin Spice Chia Pudding

Day 9:

- Breakfast: Egg and Vegetable Scramble
- Lunch: Greek Salad with Chicken

- Dinner: Turkey and Sweet Potato Casserole
- Snack: Carrot and Celery Sticks with Greek Tzatziki
- Dessert: Coconut Flour Banana Bread

Day 10:

- Breakfast: Overnight Oats with Nuts and Seeds
- Lunch: Zucchini Noodles with Pesto and Cherry Tomatoes
- Dinner: Eggplant Parmesan with Whole Wheat Pasta
- Snack: Roasted Red Pepper and Feta Dip
- Dessert: Raspberry Sorbet

Day 11:

- Breakfast: Sweet Potato and Black Bean Breakfast Hash
- Lunch: Turkey and Vegetable Stir-Fry
- Dinner: Lemon Garlic Roasted Chicken Thighs
- Snack: Avocado and Tomato Salsa
- Dessert: Nut and Seed Energy Balls

Day 12:

- Breakfast: Cottage Cheese and Pineapple Bowl

- Lunch: Caprese Salad with Balsamic Glaze
- Dinner: Blackened Salmon with Avocado Salsa
- Snack: Hard-Boiled Eggs with Mustard
- Dessert: Lemon Poppy Seed Cake (Sugar-Free)

Day 13:

- Breakfast: Almond Flour Waffles
- Lunch: Broccoli and Cheddar Stuffed Chicken Breast
- Dinner: Spaghetti Squash with Turkey Bolognese
- Snack: Whole Grain Crackers with Cheese
- Dessert: Vanilla Chia Seed Pudding with Fresh Mango

Day 14:

- Breakfast: Breakfast Burrito with Turkey Sausage
- Lunch: Whole Wheat Pasta with Tomato Sauce and Grilled Chicken
- Dinner: Chicken and Vegetable Curry
- Snack: Mini Caprese Skewers
- Dessert: Strawberry Shortcake with Almond Flour Biscuits

Day 15:

- Breakfast: Smoked Salmon and Cream Cheese Bagel
- Lunch: Vegetable and Quinoa Stuffed Peppers
- Dinner: Stuffed Portobello Mushrooms
- Snack: Smoked Salmon Cucumber Bites
- Dessert: Grilled Pineapple with Cinnamon

Day 16:

- Breakfast: Quinoa Breakfast Bowl
- Lunch: Grilled Chicken Salad with Vinaigrette
- Dinner: Baked Cod with Lemon and Herbs
- Snack: Hummus and Veggie Sticks
- Dessert: Sugar-Free Blueberry Muffins

Day 17:

- Breakfast: Veggie Omelette with Whole Grain Toast
- Lunch: Lentil and Vegetable Soup
- Dinner: Sweet Potato and Chickpea Curry
- Snack: Greek Yogurt Dip with Cucumber Slices
- Dessert: Dark Chocolate-Dipped Strawberries

Day 18:

- Breakfast: Greek Yogurt Parfait with Berries
- Lunch: Turkey and Avocado Wrap
- Dinner: Grilled Vegetable and Chicken Kebabs
- Snack: Baked Kale Chips
- Dessert: Baked Apples with Cinnamon

Day 19:

- Breakfast: Spinach and Feta Breakfast Wrap
- Lunch: Quinoa and Black Bean Bowl
- Dinner: Spinach and Mushroom Stuffed Pork Tenderloin
- Snack: Apple Slices with Almond Butter
- Dessert: Berry and Yogurt Popsicles

Day 20:

- Breakfast: Chia Seed Pudding with Almond Milk
- Lunch: Salmon and Asparagus Foil Pack
- Dinner: Beef and Broccoli Stir-Fry
- Snack: Guacamole with Whole Grain Pita Chips
- Dessert: Almond Flour Chocolate Chip Cookies

Day 21:

- Breakfast: Whole Grain Pancakes with Sugar-Free Syrup
- Lunch: Chickpea and Spinach Stew
- Dinner: Cauliflower Crust Pizza with Vegetables
- Snack: Cottage Cheese with Pineapple Chunks
- Dessert: Greek Yogurt and Berry Parfait

Week 4:

Day 22:

- Breakfast: Avocado and Tomato Breakfast Sandwich
- Lunch: Tuna Salad Lettuce Wraps
- Dinner: Quinoa-Stuffed Acorn Squash
- Snack: Mixed Nuts and Seeds Trail Mix
- Dessert: Avocado Chocolate Mousse

Day 23:

- Breakfast: Berry and Spinach Smoothie Bowl
- Lunch: Cauliflower Fried Rice with Shrimp
- Dinner: Shrimp and Vegetable Skewers
- Snack: Edamame with Sea Salt
- Dessert: Pumpkin Spice Chia Pudding

Day 24:

- Breakfast: Egg and Vegetable Scramble
- Lunch: Greek Salad with Chicken
- Dinner: Turkey and Sweet Potato Casserole
- Snack: Carrot and Celery Sticks with Greek Tzatziki
- Dessert: Coconut Flour Banana Bread

Day 25:

- Breakfast: Overnight Oats with Nuts and Seeds
- Lunch: Zucchini Noodles with Pesto and Cherry Tomatoes
- Dinner: Eggplant Parmesan with Whole Wheat Pasta
- Snack: Roasted Red Pepper and Feta Dip
- Dessert: Raspberry Sorbet

Day 26:

- Breakfast: Sweet Potato and Black Bean Breakfast Hash
- Lunch: Turkey and Vegetable Stir-Fry
- Dinner: Lemon Garlic Roasted Chicken Thighs
- Snack: Avocado and Tomato Salsa
- Dessert: Nut and Seed Energy Balls

Day 27:

- Breakfast: Cottage Cheese and Pineapple Bowl
- Lunch: Caprese Salad with Balsamic Glaze
- Dinner: Blackened Salmon with Avocado Salsa
- Snack: Hard-Boiled Eggs with Mustard
- Dessert: Lemon Poppy Seed Cake (Sugar-Free)

Day 28:

- Breakfast: Almond Flour Waffles
- Lunch: Broccoli and Cheddar Stuffed Chicken Breast
- Dinner: Spaghetti Squash with Turkey Bolognese
- Snack: Whole Grain Crackers with Cheese
- Dessert: Vanilla Chia Seed Pudding with Fresh Mango

Day 29:

- Breakfast: Breakfast Burrito with Turkey Sausage
- Lunch: Whole Wheat Pasta with Tomato Sauce and Grilled Chicken
- Dinner: Chicken and Vegetable Curry
- Snack: Mini Caprese Skewers

- Dessert: Strawberry Shortcake with Almond Flour Biscuits

Day 30:

- Breakfast: Smoked Salmon and Cream Cheese Bagel
- Lunch: Vegetable and Quinoa Stuffed Peppers
- Dinner: Stuffed Portobello Mushrooms
- Snack: Smoked Salmon Cucumber Bites
- Dessert: Grilled Pineapple with Cinnamon

Chapter 2: Breakfast Recipes

These recipes are crafted with a fusion of flavors and nutritional goodness, ensuring a balance of essential nutrients to kickstart your day. Each recipe is not only a culinary delight but also a thoughtful selection to help regulate blood sugar levels.

Quinoa Breakfast Bowl

Ingredients:

- 1/2 cup cooked quinoa
- 1/4 cup fresh blueberries
- 1 tablespoon chopped walnuts
- 1 teaspoon honey
- 1/2 teaspoon cinnamon

Instructions:

1. In a bowl, combine cooked quinoa, fresh blueberries, and chopped walnuts.
2. Drizzle honey over the mixture and sprinkle with cinnamon.

3. Stir well and savor the nutritious blend.

Nutrition Information (per serving):

- Calories: 250
- Protein: 8g
- Carbohydrates: 40g
- Fat: 8g
- Fiber: 6g
- Sugar: 8g
- Portion Size: 1 bowl

Veggie Omelette with Whole Grain Toast

Ingredients:

- 2 large eggs
- 1/4 cup diced bell peppers
- 1/4 cup diced tomatoes
- 1/4 cup chopped spinach
- Salt and pepper to taste
- 1 slice whole grain bread, toasted

Instructions:

1. Whisk eggs in a bowl and season with salt and pepper.
2. In a non-stick pan, sauté bell peppers, tomatoes, and spinach until tender.
3. Pour whisked eggs over the veggies, cook until set, and fold into an omelette.
4. Serve with a slice of toasted whole grain bread.

Nutrition Information (per serving):

- Calories: 280
- Protein: 15g
- Carbohydrates: 20g
- Fat: 16g
- Fiber: 5g
- Sugar: 3g
- Portion Size: 1 omelette with toast

Greek Yogurt Parfait with Berries

Ingredients:

- 1/2 cup Greek yogurt

- 1/4 cup mixed berries (strawberries, blueberries, raspberries)
- 1 tablespoon almond slices
- 1 teaspoon honey

Instructions:

1. In a glass, layer Greek yogurt with mixed berries.
2. Sprinkle almond slices over each layer.
3. Drizzle honey on top for sweetness.

Nutrition Information (per serving):

- Calories: 180
- Protein: 15g
- Carbohydrates: 20g
- Fat: 7g
- Fiber: 4g
- Sugar: 12g
- Portion Size: 1 parfait

Spinach and Feta Breakfast Wrap

Ingredients:

- 1 whole wheat tortilla

- 2 large eggs, scrambled
- 1/4 cup fresh spinach, chopped
- 2 tablespoons crumbled feta cheese
- Salt and pepper to taste

Instructions:

1. Scramble eggs in a pan, season with salt and pepper.
2. Lay the tortilla flat and assemble with eggs, chopped spinach, and feta.
3. Roll into a wrap and enjoy!

Nutrition Information (per serving):

- Calories: 320
- Protein: 18g
- Carbohydrates: 24g
- Fat: 18g
- Fiber: 5g
- Sugar: 2g
- Portion Size: 1 wrap

Chia Seed Pudding with Almond Milk

Ingredients:

- 2 tablespoons chia seeds
- 1/2 cup unsweetened almond milk
- 1/4 teaspoon vanilla extract
- Fresh berries for topping

Instructions:

1. Mix chia seeds, almond milk, and vanilla extract in a jar.
2. Stir well, refrigerate for at least 2 hours or overnight.
3. Top with fresh berries before serving.

Nutrition Information (per serving):

- Calories: 120
- Protein: 4g
- Carbohydrates: 12g
- Fat: 7g
- Fiber: 8g
- Sugar: 2g
- Portion Size: 1 pudding

Whole Grain Pancakes with Sugar-Free Syrup

Ingredients:

- 1/2 cup whole wheat flour
- 1/2 teaspoon baking powder
- 1/4 teaspoon cinnamon
- 1/2 cup almond milk
- 1 tablespoon unsweetened applesauce
- Sugar-free syrup for topping

Instructions:

1. Mix whole wheat flour, baking powder, and cinnamon.
2. Add almond milk and applesauce, stir until smooth.
3. Cook pancakes on a griddle and serve with sugar-free syrup.

Nutrition Information (per serving):

- Calories: 220
- Protein: 8g
- Carbohydrates: 40g
- Fat: 3g

- Fiber: 6g

- Sugar: 2g

- Portion Size: 3 pancakes

Avocado and Tomato Breakfast Sandwich

Ingredients:

- 1 whole grain English muffin, toasted

- 1/2 avocado, mashed

- 1 medium tomato, sliced

- Salt and pepper to taste

Instructions:

1. Toast the English muffin to your liking.
2. Spread mashed avocado on each half.
3. Top with sliced tomatoes and season with salt and pepper.

Nutrition Information (per serving):

- Calories: 280

- Protein: 7g

- Carbohydrates: 32g
- Fat: 16g
- Fiber: 8g
- Sugar: 3g
- Portion Size: 1 sandwich

Berry and Spinach Smoothie Bowl

Ingredients:

- 1 cup fresh spinach
- 1/2 cup mixed berries (strawberries, blueberries, raspberries)
- 1/2 banana, frozen
- 1/2 cup unsweetened almond milk
- Toppings: Granola, sliced almonds, chia seeds

Instructions:

1. Blend spinach, berries, banana, and almond milk until smooth.
2. Pour into a bowl and top with granola, sliced almonds, and chia seeds.

Nutrition Information (per serving):

- Calories: 220
- Protein: 6g
- Carbohydrates: 40g
- Fat: 5g
- Fiber: 8g
- Sugar: 14g
- Portion Size: 1 bowl

Egg and Vegetable Scramble

Ingredients:

- 2 large eggs
- 1/4 cup diced bell peppers
- 1/4 cup diced zucchini
- 1/4 cup cherry tomatoes, halved
- Fresh herbs for garnish

Instructions:

1. Whisk eggs and season with salt and pepper.
2. In a pan, sauté bell peppers, zucchini, and cherry tomatoes.

3. Add whisked eggs and scramble until cooked. Garnish with fresh herbs.

Nutrition Information (per serving):

- Calories: 210
- Protein: 14g
- Carbohydrates: 12g
- Fat: 12g
- Fiber: 3g
- Sugar: 5g
- Portion Size: 1 serving

Overnight Oats with Nuts and Seeds

Ingredients:

- 1/2 cup rolled oats
- 1/2 cup unsweetened almond milk
- 1 tablespoon chia seeds
- 1 tablespoon chopped nuts (almonds, walnuts)
- 1/2 teaspoon vanilla extract

Instructions:

1. Mix oats, almond milk, chia seeds, chopped nuts, and vanilla extract in a jar.

2. Refrigerate overnight and enjoy in the morning.

Nutrition Information (per serving):

- Calories: 280
- Protein: 10g
- Carbohydrates: 35g
- Fat: 12g
- Fiber: 8g
- Sugar: 3g
- Portion Size: 1 jar

Sweet Potato and Black Bean Breakfast Hash

Ingredients:

- 1 medium sweet potato, diced
- 1/2 cup black beans, canned and rinsed
- 1/4 cup red onion, diced
- 1 teaspoon olive oil

- 1/2 teaspoon cumin

- Salt and pepper to taste

Instructions:

1. In a pan, sauté sweet potatoes, black beans, and red onion in olive oil.
2. Season with cumin, salt, and pepper.
3. Cook until sweet potatoes are tender. Serve hot.

Nutrition Information (per serving):

- Calories: 240

- Protein: 8g

- Carbohydrates: 45g

- Fat: 3g

- Fiber: 10g

- Sugar: 6g

- Portion Size: 1 serving

Cottage Cheese and Pineapple Bowl

Ingredients:

- 1/2 cup low-fat cottage cheese

- 1/2 cup fresh pineapple chunks

- 1 tablespoon shredded coconut

Instructions:

1. Combine cottage cheese and pineapple chunks in a bowl.
2. Sprinkle shredded coconut on top.
3. Mix gently and enjoy this tropical delight.

Nutrition Information (per serving):

- Calories: 180
- Protein: 15g
- Carbohydrates: 25g
- Fat: 3g
- Fiber: 3g
- Sugar: 20g
- Portion Size: 1 bowl

Almond Flour Waffles

Ingredients:

- 1 cup almond flour
- 2 eggs
- 1/4 cup almond milk

- 1 tablespoon coconut oil, melted
- 1/2 teaspoon baking powder

Instructions:

1. Mix almond flour, eggs, almond milk, melted coconut oil, and baking powder.
2. Pour batter into a preheated waffle iron and cook until golden brown.
3. Serve with your favorite toppings.

Nutrition Information (per serving):

- Calories: 290
- Protein: 12g
- Carbohydrates: 8g
- Fat: 25g
- Fiber: 4g
- Sugar: 2g
- Portion Size: 2 waffles

Breakfast Burrito with Turkey Sausage

Ingredients:

- 1 whole wheat tortilla
- 2 turkey sausage links, cooked
- 1/4 cup black beans, canned and rinsed
- 1/4 cup shredded cheese
- Salsa for topping

Instructions:

1. Lay out the tortilla and assemble with turkey sausage, black beans, and shredded cheese.
2. Roll into a burrito and heat in a pan until the cheese melts.
3. Top with salsa before serving.

Nutrition Information (per serving):

- Calories: 320
- Protein: 18g
- Carbohydrates: 25g
- Fat: 16g
- Fiber: 6g

- Sugar: 2g
- Portion Size: 1 burrito

Smoked Salmon and Cream Cheese Bagel

Ingredients:

- 1 whole grain bagel, toasted
- 2 tablespoons cream cheese
- 2 ounces smoked salmon
- Capers and fresh dill for garnish

Instructions:

1. Toast the whole grain bagel to your liking.
2. Spread cream cheese on each half.
3. Top with smoked salmon, capers, and fresh dill.

Nutrition Information (per serving):

- Calories: 280
- Protein: 15g
- Carbohydrates: 35g
- Fat: 10g

- Fiber: 6g
- Sugar: 2g
- Portion Size: 1 bagel

Chapter 3: Lunch Recipes

These carefully crafted meals are designed to not only tantalize your taste buds but also support your health goals by managing blood sugar levels. Each recipe is a testament to the idea that eating well can be both a pleasure and a path to wellness.

Grilled Chicken Salad with Vinaigrette

Ingredients:

- 1 boneless, skinless chicken breast
- Mixed salad greens (spinach, arugula, and romaine)
- Cherry tomatoes, halved
- Cucumber, sliced
- Red bell pepper, thinly sliced
- Balsamic vinaigrette dressing

Instructions:

1. Grill the chicken breast until fully cooked.
2. Slice the grilled chicken into strips.

3. In a large bowl, combine salad greens, cherry tomatoes, cucumber, and red bell pepper.

4. Top the salad with grilled chicken strips.

5. Drizzle balsamic vinaigrette over the salad.

6. Toss gently to combine.

Nutrition Information (per serving):

- Calories: 350
- Protein: 28g
- Carbohydrates: 15g
- Fat: 18g
- Fiber: 5g
- Sugar: 7g
- Portion Size: 1 serving

Lentil and Vegetable Soup

Ingredients:

- 1 cup dried lentils, rinsed
- Carrots, chopped
- Celery, chopped
- Onion, diced
- Garlic, minced

- Vegetable broth
- Cumin, ground
- Paprika
- Salt and pepper to taste

Instructions:

1. In a large pot, sauté onions and garlic until translucent.
2. Add lentils, carrots, celery, and vegetable broth to the pot.
3. Season with cumin, paprika, salt, and pepper.
4. Bring to a boil, then reduce heat and simmer until lentils are tender.

Nutrition Information (per serving):

- Calories: 220
- Protein: 14g
- Carbohydrates: 40g
- Fat: 1g
- Fiber: 15g
- Sugar: 5g
- Portion Size: 1 cup

Turkey and Avocado Wrap

Ingredients:

- Whole grain wrap
- Sliced turkey breast
- Avocado, sliced
- Lettuce leaves
- Tomato, sliced
- Mustard or low-fat mayo (optional)

Instructions:

1. Lay out the whole grain wrap.
2. Layer sliced turkey, avocado, lettuce, and tomato.
3. Add mustard or low-fat mayo if desired.
4. Roll the wrap tightly and cut in half.

Nutrition Information (per serving):

- Calories: 320
- Protein: 22g
- Carbohydrates: 35g
- Fat: 12g
- Fiber: 8g
- Sugar: 3g

- Portion Size: 1 wrap

Quinoa and Black Bean Bowl

Ingredients:

- Cooked quinoa
- Black beans, rinsed and drained
- Corn kernels
- Red onion, finely chopped
- Avocado, diced
- Fresh cilantro, chopped
- Lime juice
- Olive oil
- Salt and pepper to taste

Instructions:

1. In a bowl, combine cooked quinoa, black beans, corn, red onion, and diced avocado.
2. In a small bowl, whisk together lime juice, olive oil, salt, and pepper.
3. Pour the dressing over the quinoa mixture and toss gently.

Nutrition Information (per serving):

- Calories: 380
- Protein: 15g
- Carbohydrates: 55g
- Fat: 14g
- Fiber: 12g
- Sugar: 3g
- Portion Size: 1 cup

Salmon and Asparagus Foil Pack

Ingredients:

- Salmon fillet
- Asparagus spears
- Lemon slices
- Garlic, minced
- Dill, chopped
- Olive oil
- Salt and pepper to taste

Instructions:

1. Preheat the oven to 400°F (200°C).
2. Place a salmon fillet on a sheet of foil.

3. Arrange asparagus around the salmon, add lemon slices, and sprinkle with minced garlic and chopped dill.

4. Drizzle with olive oil, season with salt and pepper, then seal the foil.

5. Bake for 15-20 minutes or until salmon is cooked through.

Nutrition Information (per serving):

- Calories: 320
- Protein: 30g
- Carbohydrates: 8g
- Fat: 18g
- Fiber: 3g
- Sugar: 2g
- Portion Size: 1 foil pack

Chickpea and Spinach Stew

Ingredients:

- Chickpeas, canned and drained
- Spinach leaves
- Tomatoes, diced

- Onion, finely chopped

- Garlic, minced

- Vegetable broth

- Cumin, ground

- Paprika

- Salt and pepper to taste

Instructions:

1. In a pot, sauté onions and garlic until softened.

2. Add chickpeas, spinach, diced tomatoes, and vegetable broth.

3. Season with cumin, paprika, salt, and pepper.

4. Simmer until spinach is wilted and flavors meld.

Nutrition Information (per serving):

- Calories: 280

- Protein: 14g

- Carbohydrates: 45g

- Fat: 5g

- Fiber: 12g

- Sugar: 8g

- Portion Size: 1 cup

Tuna Salad Lettuce Wraps

Ingredients:

- Canned tuna, drained
- Greek yogurt
- Celery, finely chopped
- Red onion, minced
- Dill pickles, diced
- Lettuce leaves for wrapping

Instructions:

1. In a bowl, mix tuna, Greek yogurt, celery, red onion, and dill pickles.
2. Spoon the tuna salad onto lettuce leaves.
3. Roll the lettuce leaves to create wraps.

Nutrition Information (per serving):

- Calories: 240
- Protein: 20g
- Carbohydrates: 10g
- Fat: 12g
- Fiber: 3g
- Sugar: 3g

- Portion Size: 2 wraps

Cauliflower Fried Rice with Shrimp

Ingredients:

- Cauliflower rice
- Shrimp, peeled and deveined
- Mixed vegetables (peas, carrots, corn)
- Eggs, beaten
- Soy sauce
- Sesame oil
- Green onions, chopped
- Garlic, minced

Instructions:

1. In a wok or large skillet, sauté shrimp, garlic, and mixed vegetables.
2. Push ingredients to the side, pour beaten eggs into the empty space, and scramble.
3. Add cauliflower rice, soy sauce, and sesame oil.
4. Stir-fry until cauliflower is tender.
5. Garnish with chopped green onions.

Nutrition Information (per serving):

- Calories: 280
- Protein: 22g
- Carbohydrates: 20g
- Fat: 12g
- Fiber: 6g
- Sugar: 5g
- Portion Size: 1.5 cups

Greek Salad with Chicken

Ingredients:

- Grilled chicken breast, sliced
- Mixed salad greens
- Cherry tomatoes, halved
- Cucumber, sliced
- Kalamata olives, pitted
- Feta cheese, crumbled
- Greek dressing

Instructions:

1. Arrange salad greens on a plate.

2. Top with sliced grilled chicken, cherry tomatoes, cucumber, olives, and feta cheese.

3. Drizzle with Greek dressing.

Nutrition Information (per serving):

- Calories: 320

- Protein: 28g

- Carbohydrates: 10g

- Fat: 18g

- Fiber: 4g

- Sugar: 5g

- Portion Size: 1.5 cups

Zucchini Noodles with Pesto and Cherry Tomatoes

Ingredients:

- Zucchini, spiralized into noodles

- Cherry tomatoes, halved

- Pesto sauce (homemade or store-bought)

- Parmesan cheese, grated

- Pine nuts (optional)

Instructions:

1. Sauté zucchini noodles in a pan until slightly softened.
2. Toss with cherry tomatoes and pesto sauce.
3. Sprinkle with grated Parmesan cheese and pine nuts.

Nutrition Information (per serving):

- Calories: 250
- Protein: 8g
- Carbohydrates: 15g
- Fat: 18g
- Fiber: 5g
- Sugar: 7g
- Portion Size: 1.5 cups

Turkey and Vegetable Stir-Fry

Ingredients:

- Turkey breast, thinly sliced
- Broccoli florets
- Bell peppers, sliced
- Snow peas
- Ginger, minced

- Garlic, minced

- Low-sodium soy sauce

- Sesame oil

- Brown rice, cooked

Instructions:

1. In a wok or skillet, stir-fry turkey until cooked through.
2. Add broccoli, bell peppers, snow peas, ginger, and garlic.
3. Drizzle with soy sauce and sesame oil.
4. Continue stir-frying until vegetables are tender-crisp.
5. Serve over cooked brown rice.

Nutrition Information (per serving):

- Calories: 340

- Protein: 30g

- Carbohydrates: 40g

- Fat: 8g

- Fiber: 7g

- Sugar: 5g

- Portion Size: 1 cup stir-fry with 1/2 cup rice

Caprese Salad with Balsamic Glaze

Ingredients:

- Tomatoes, sliced
- Fresh mozzarella, sliced
- Fresh basil leaves
- Balsamic glaze
- Olive oil
- Salt and pepper to taste

Instructions:

1. Arrange alternating slices of tomatoes and mozzarella on a plate.
2. Tuck fresh basil leaves between tomato and mozzarella slices.
3. Drizzle with balsamic glaze and olive oil.
4. Season with salt and pepper.

Nutrition Information (per serving):

- Calories: 280
- Protein: 14g
- Carbohydrates: 10g
- Fat: 20g

- Fiber: 2g

- Sugar: 6g

- Portion Size: 1.5 cups

Broccoli and Cheddar Stuffed Chicken Breast

Ingredients:

- Chicken breast, boneless and skinless

- Broccoli florets, steamed

- Cheddar cheese, shredded

- Garlic powder

- Paprika

- Salt and pepper to taste

Instructions:

1. Preheat the oven to 375°F (190°C).

2. Cut a pocket into each chicken breast.

3. Stuff with steamed broccoli and cheddar cheese.

4. Season the outside with garlic powder, paprika, salt, and pepper.

5. Bake until chicken is cooked through.

Nutrition Information (per serving):

- Calories: 320
- Protein: 40g
- Carbohydrates: 6g
- Fat: 15g
- Fiber: 3g
- Sugar: 2g
- Portion Size: 1 stuffed chicken breast

Whole Wheat Pasta with Tomato Sauce and Grilled Chicken

Ingredients:

- Whole wheat pasta, cooked
- Grilled chicken breast, sliced
- Tomatoes, diced
- Garlic, minced
- Olive oil
- Basil, chopped
- Parmesan cheese, grated

Instructions:

1. In a pan, sauté garlic in olive oil until fragrant.

2. Add diced tomatoes and cook until softened.

3. Toss in cooked whole wheat pasta and grilled chicken.

4. Sprinkle with chopped basil and grated Parmesan.

Nutrition Information (per serving):

- Calories: 380
- Protein: 30g
- Carbohydrates: 40g
- Fat: 12g
- Fiber: 8g
- Sugar: 4g
- Portion Size: 1.5 cups

Vegetable and Quinoa Stuffed Peppers

Ingredients:

- Bell peppers, halved and seeds removed
- Quinoa, cooked

- Black beans, rinsed and drained

- Corn kernels

- Onion, diced

- Tomato sauce

- Cumin, ground

- Chili powder

- Shredded cheese (optional)

Instructions:

1. Preheat the oven to 375°F (190°C).

2. In a bowl, mix cooked quinoa, black beans, corn, diced onion, tomato sauce, cumin, and chili powder.

3. Spoon the mixture into halved bell peppers.

4. If desired, sprinkle with shredded cheese.

5. Bake until peppers are tender.

Nutrition Information (per serving):

- Calories: 310

- Protein: 15g

- Carbohydrates: 50g

- Fat: 7g

- Fiber: 12g

- Sugar: 8g

- Portion Size: 2 stuffed pepper halves

Chapter 4: Dinner Recipes

These recipes are thoughtfully designed to incorporate a variety of ingredients that bring together the perfect balance of taste and nutrition. Each dish is not only a feast for the senses but also a nourishing choice for managing blood sugar levels.

Baked Cod with Lemon and Herbs

Ingredients:

- 4 cod fillets
- 2 tablespoons olive oil
- 1 lemon (juiced and zest)
- 2 cloves garlic (minced)
- 1 teaspoon dried thyme
- Salt and pepper to taste

Instructions:

1. Preheat the oven to 375°F (190°C).
2. Place cod fillets on a baking sheet.

3. Mix olive oil, lemon juice, lemon zest, garlic, thyme, salt, and pepper in a bowl.

4. Brush the mixture over the cod fillets.

5. Bake for 15-20 minutes or until the cod is cooked through.

6. Serve hot, garnished with fresh herbs.

Nutrition Information (per serving):

- Calories: 250
- Protein: 30g
- Carbohydrates: 3g
- Fat: 12g
- Fiber: 1g
- Sugar: 0g
- Portion Size: 1 fillet

Sweet Potato and Chickpea Curry

Ingredients:

- 2 sweet potatoes (peeled and diced)
- 1 can chickpeas (drained)
- 1 onion (chopped)
- 2 cloves garlic (minced)

- 1 can coconut milk

- 2 tablespoons curry powder

- Salt and pepper to taste

Instructions:

1. In a pan, sauté onion and garlic until softened.

2. Add sweet potatoes, chickpeas, coconut milk, curry powder, salt, and pepper.

3. Simmer until sweet potatoes are tender.

4. Serve over brown rice or quinoa.

Nutrition Information (per serving):

- Calories: 320

- Protein: 8g

- Carbohydrates: 45g

- Fat: 14g

- Fiber: 10g

- Sugar: 8g

- Portion Size: 1 cup

Grilled Vegetable and Chicken Kebabs

Ingredients:

- 1 lb chicken breast (cubed)
- Assorted vegetables (bell peppers, zucchini, cherry tomatoes)
- 2 tablespoons olive oil
- 1 teaspoon dried oregano
- 1 teaspoon paprika
- Salt and pepper to taste

Instructions:

1. Thread chicken and vegetables onto skewers.
2. Mix olive oil, oregano, paprika, salt, and pepper.
3. Brush the mixture over the kebabs.
4. Grill until chicken is cooked and vegetables are tender.
5. Serve hot with a side salad.

Nutrition Information (per serving):

- Calories: 280
- Protein: 30g

- Carbohydrates: 10g

- Fat: 12g

- Fiber: 3g

- Sugar: 4g

- Portion Size: 2 kebabs

Spinach and Mushroom Stuffed Pork Tenderloin

Ingredients:

- 1 pork tenderloin

- 2 cups fresh spinach

- 1 cup mushrooms (sliced)

- 2 cloves garlic (minced)

- 1 tablespoon olive oil

- 1 teaspoon dried thyme

- Salt and pepper to taste

Instructions:

1. Preheat the oven to 400°F (200°C).

2. Butterfly the pork tenderloin.

3. Sauté spinach, mushrooms, and garlic in olive oil.

4. Spread the mixture over the pork, roll, and secure with toothpicks.

5. Season with thyme, salt, and pepper.

6. Roast for 25-30 minutes or until cooked.

7. Slice and serve.

Nutrition Information (per serving):

- Calories: 290
- Protein: 35g
- Carbohydrates: 4g
- Fat: 15g
- Fiber: 2g
- Sugar: 1g
- Portion Size: 1 slice

Beef and Broccoli Stir-Fry

Ingredients:

- 1 lb lean beef strips
- 2 cups broccoli florets
- 1 bell pepper (sliced)
- 3 tablespoons low-sodium soy sauce
- 1 tablespoon sesame oil

- 1 tablespoon ginger (minced)
- 2 cloves garlic (minced)

Instructions:

1. In a wok, stir-fry beef until browned. Set aside.
2. Stir-fry broccoli, bell pepper, ginger, and garlic in sesame oil.
3. Add cooked beef back to the wok.
4. Pour soy sauce over the mixture and toss until well-coated.
5. Serve over cauliflower rice.

Nutrition Information (per serving):

- Calories: 310
- Protein: 28g
- Carbohydrates: 10g
- Fat: 18g
- Fiber: 3g
- Sugar: 3g
- Portion Size: 1 cup

Cauliflower Crust Pizza with Vegetables

Ingredients:

- 1 cauliflower crust (store-bought or homemade)
- 1/2 cup tomato sauce (sugar-free)
- 1 cup assorted vegetables (bell peppers, cherry tomatoes, mushrooms)
- 1 cup part-skim mozzarella cheese
- 1 teaspoon dried basil
- 1 teaspoon dried oregano

Instructions:

1. Preheat the oven according to the cauliflower crust instructions.
2. Spread tomato sauce over the crust.
3. Top with vegetables and mozzarella cheese.
4. Sprinkle with basil and oregano.
5. Bake until the crust is golden and the cheese is melted.

Nutrition Information (per serving):

- Calories: 220

- Protein: 15g

- Carbohydrates: 15g

- Fat: 12g

- Fiber: 5g

- Sugar: 3g

- Portion Size: 1/4 pizza

Quinoa-Stuffed Acorn Squash

Ingredients:

- 2 acorn squash (halved and seeded)

- 1 cup cooked quinoa

- 1 cup black beans (canned, drained)

- 1 cup diced tomatoes

- 1 teaspoon cumin

- 1 teaspoon chili powder

- Salt and pepper to taste

Instructions:

1. Preheat the oven to 375°F (190°C).

2. Place acorn squash halves on a baking sheet.

3. In a bowl, mix cooked quinoa, black beans, diced tomatoes, cumin, chili powder, salt, and pepper.

4. Stuff each squash half with the quinoa mixture.

5. Bake for 25-30 minutes or until squash is tender.

Nutrition Information (per serving):

- Calories: 280
- Protein: 12g
- Carbohydrates: 55g
- Fat: 2g
- Fiber: 10g
- Sugar: 4g
- Portion Size: 1/2 squash

Shrimp and Vegetable Skewers

Ingredients:

- 1 lb shrimp (peeled and deveined)
- Assorted vegetables (bell peppers, cherry tomatoes, red onions)
- 2 tablespoons olive oil
- 1 teaspoon garlic powder
- 1 teaspoon paprika
- Salt and pepper to taste

Instructions:

1. Preheat the grill or oven to medium-high heat.
2. Thread shrimp and vegetables onto skewers.
3. Mix olive oil, garlic powder, paprika, salt, and pepper.
4. Brush the mixture over the skewers.
5. Grill or bake until shrimp is opaque and vegetables are tender.
6. Serve hot with a squeeze of lemon.

Nutrition Information (per serving):

- Calories: 210
- Protein: 25g
- Carbohydrates: 8g
- Fat: 8g
- Fiber: 2g
- Sugar: 3g
- Portion Size: 2 skewers

Turkey and Sweet Potato Casserole

Ingredients:

- 1 lb ground turkey

- 2 sweet potatoes (peeled and sliced)
- 1 cup low-sodium chicken broth
- 1 cup green beans (trimmed)
- 1 onion (chopped)
- 2 cloves garlic (minced)
- 1 teaspoon dried thyme
- Salt and pepper to taste

Instructions:

1. Preheat the oven to 375°F (190°C).
2. In a skillet, brown ground turkey with garlic and onion.
3. Layer sweet potatoes and green beans in a casserole dish.
4. Pour chicken broth over the vegetables.
5. Spread the turkey mixture on top.
6. Sprinkle with thyme, salt, and pepper.
7. Cover and bake for 30-40 minutes or until sweet potatoes are tender.

Nutrition Information (per serving):

- Calories: 290

- Protein: 25g

- Carbohydrates: 25g

- Fat: 10g

- Fiber: 5g

- Sugar: 6g

- Portion Size: 1 cup

Eggplant Parmesan with Whole Wheat Pasta

Ingredients:

- 1 large eggplant (sliced)

- 1 cup whole wheat pasta

- 2 cups marinara sauce (low-sugar)

- 1 cup part-skim mozzarella cheese

- 1/2 cup grated Parmesan cheese

- 1 teaspoon dried basil

- 1 teaspoon dried oregano

Instructions:

1. Preheat the oven to 375°F (190°C).

2. Bake eggplant slices until tender.

3. Cook whole wheat pasta according to package instructions.

4. In a baking dish, layer marinara sauce, eggplant, pasta, and cheeses.

5. Repeat layers, finishing with a cheese layer on top.

6. Sprinkle with basil and oregano.

7. Bake for 25-30 minutes or until bubbly and golden.

Nutrition Information (per serving):

- Calories: 320
- Protein: 15g
- Carbohydrates: 35g
- Fat: 14g
- Fiber: 8g
- Sugar: 5g
- Portion Size: 1 cup

Lemon Garlic Roasted Chicken Thighs

Ingredients:

- 4 chicken thighs (bone-in, skin-on)

- 1 lemon (juiced and zest)
- 3 cloves garlic (minced)
- 2 tablespoons olive oil
- 1 teaspoon dried rosemary
- Salt and pepper to taste

Instructions:

1. Preheat the oven to 400°F (200°C).
2. In a bowl, mix lemon juice, lemon zest, minced garlic, olive oil, rosemary, salt, and pepper.
3. Place chicken thighs in a baking dish and brush the mixture over them.
4. Roast for 35-40 minutes or until the chicken is golden and cooked through.
5. Serve hot, garnished with fresh herbs.

Nutrition Information (per serving):

- Calories: 280
- Protein: 25g
- Carbohydrates: 2g
- Fat: 18g
- Fiber: 0g

- Sugar: 1g

- Portion Size: 1 thigh

Blackened Salmon with Avocado Salsa

Ingredients:

- 4 salmon fillets

- 1 tablespoon blackened seasoning

- 2 avocados (diced)

- 1 cup cherry tomatoes (halved)

- 1/4 cup red onion (finely chopped)

- 1/4 cup fresh cilantro (chopped)

- 1 lime (juiced)

- Salt and pepper to taste

Instructions:

1. Rub blackened seasoning over salmon fillets.

2. In a bowl, combine diced avocados, cherry tomatoes, red onion, cilantro, lime juice, salt, and pepper to make the salsa.

3. Grill or bake salmon until cooked through.

4. Top salmon with avocado salsa before serving.

Nutrition Information (per serving):

- Calories: 320
- Protein: 28g
- Carbohydrates: 12g
- Fat: 18g
- Fiber: 6g
- Sugar: 2g
- Portion Size: 1 fillet

Spaghetti Squash with Turkey Bolognese

Ingredients:

- 1 large spaghetti squash
- 1 lb ground turkey
- 2 cups tomato sauce (low-sugar)
- 1 onion (chopped)
- 2 cloves garlic (minced)
- 1 teaspoon dried Italian herbs
- Salt and pepper to taste

Instructions:

1. Preheat the oven to 375°F (190°C).

2. Cut spaghetti squash in half, scoop out seeds, and bake until fork-tender.

3. In a skillet, brown ground turkey with garlic and onion.

4. Add tomato sauce, Italian herbs, salt, and pepper to the turkey.

5. Use a fork to scrape the cooked spaghetti squash into "noodles."

6. Top with turkey bolognese and serve.

Nutrition Information (per serving):

- Calories: 280
- Protein: 22g
- Carbohydrates: 20g
- Fat: 12g
- Fiber: 5g
- Sugar: 7g
- Portion Size: 1 cup

Chicken and Vegetable Curry

Ingredients:

- 1 lb chicken breast (cubed)
- 2 cups mixed vegetables (broccoli, carrots, bell peppers)
- 1 can coconut milk
- 3 tablespoons curry powder
- 2 tablespoons olive oil
- 1 onion (chopped)
- 2 cloves garlic (minced)
- Salt and pepper to taste

Instructions:

1. In a large pan, sauté chicken, garlic, and onion in olive oil until chicken is browned.
2. Add mixed vegetables and continue to cook until vegetables are tender.
3. Pour in coconut milk and stir in curry powder, salt, and pepper.
4. Simmer until chicken is cooked through and flavors meld.
5. Serve over cauliflower rice.

Nutrition Information (per serving):

- Calories: 350
- Protein: 28g
- Carbohydrates: 15g
- Fat: 20g
- Fiber: 4g
- Sugar: 5g
- Portion Size: 1 cup

Stuffed Portobello Mushrooms

Ingredients:

- 4 large Portobello mushrooms
- 1 lb ground turkey
- 1 cup spinach (chopped)
- 1/2 cup feta cheese (crumbled)
- 2 tablespoons olive oil
- 2 cloves garlic (minced)
- Salt and pepper to taste

Instructions:

1. Preheat the oven to 375°F (190°C).

2. Remove stems from Portobello mushrooms and brush with olive oil.

3. In a skillet, sauté ground turkey, garlic, and spinach until turkey is browned.

4. Stuff each mushroom with the turkey mixture and top with crumbled feta.

5. Bake for 20-25 minutes or until mushrooms are tender.

Nutrition Information (per serving):

- Calories: 260
- Protein: 20g
- Carbohydrates: 10g
- Fat: 15g
- Fiber: 3g
- Sugar: 4g
- Portion Size: 1 mushroom

Chapter 5: Snacks and Appetizers

These recipes combine wholesome ingredients, bold flavors, and balanced nutrition to satisfy cravings without compromising health. From crunchy veggie sticks paired with creamy hummus to savory mini caprese skewers, these snacks promise a delightful journey for the palate.

Hummus and Veggie Sticks

Ingredients:

- 1 cup chickpeas (canned, drained)
- 2 cloves garlic
- 3 tbsp tahini
- 3 tbsp lemon juice
- 2 tbsp olive oil
- 1/2 tsp cumin
- Salt and pepper to taste
- Assorted veggie sticks (carrots, cucumber, bell peppers)

Instructions:

1. In a food processor, blend chickpeas, garlic, tahini, lemon juice, olive oil, cumin, salt, and pepper until smooth.
2. Serve the hummus with a variety of veggie sticks for a colorful and nutritious snack.

Nutrition Information (per serving):

- Calories: 120
- Protein: 4g
- Carbohydrates: 15g
- Fat: 6g
- Fiber: 5g
- Sugar: 2g
- Portion Size: 2 tbsp hummus with veggie sticks

Greek Yogurt Dip with Cucumber Slices

Ingredients:

- 1 cup Greek yogurt
- 1/2 cucumber, thinly sliced

- 1 tbsp fresh dill, chopped

- 1 clove garlic, minced

- Salt and pepper to taste

Instructions:

1. In a bowl, combine Greek yogurt, dill, garlic, salt, and pepper.

2. Chill the dip in the refrigerator for at least 30 minutes.

3. Serve with cucumber slices for a refreshing and protein-packed snack.

Nutrition Information (per serving):

- Calories: 80

- Protein: 10g

- Carbohydrates: 5g

- Fat: 2g

- Fiber: 1g

- Sugar: 3g

- Portion Size: 1/2 cup dip with cucumber slices

Baked Kale Chips

Ingredients:

- 1 bunch kale, stems removed and torn into bite-sized pieces
- 1 tbsp olive oil
- Salt and pepper to taste

Instructions:

1. Preheat oven to 350°F (175°C).
2. Toss kale with olive oil, salt, and pepper.
3. Arrange kale in a single layer on a baking sheet.
4. Bake for 10-15 minutes or until crisp, turning halfway through.

Nutrition Information (per serving):

- Calories: 50
- Protein: 2g
- Carbohydrates: 8g
- Fat: 2g
- Fiber: 2g
- Sugar: 1g
- Portion Size: 1 cup baked kale chips

Apple Slices with Almond Butter

Ingredients:

- 1 apple, sliced
- 2 tbsp almond butter

Instructions:

1. Spread almond butter on apple slices.
2. Enjoy this simple and satisfying combination.

Nutrition Information (per serving):

- Calories: 180
- Protein: 4g
- Carbohydrates: 19g
- Fat: 11g
- Fiber: 5g
- Sugar: 12g
- Portion Size: 1 medium apple with almond butter

Guacamole with Whole Grain Pita Chips

Ingredients:

- 2 ripe avocados, mashed
- 1 tomato, diced
- 1/4 cup red onion, finely chopped
- 1 clove garlic, minced
- 1 lime, juiced
- Salt and pepper to taste
- Whole grain pita chips

Instructions:

1. In a bowl, combine avocados, tomato, red onion, garlic, lime juice, salt, and pepper.
2. Serve with whole grain pita chips for a heart-healthy snack.

Nutrition Information (per serving):

- Calories: 160
- Protein: 3g
- Carbohydrates: 19g
- Fat: 9g

- Fiber: 7g
- Sugar: 2g
- Portion Size: 1/2 cup guacamole with 10 pita chips

Cottage Cheese with Pineapple Chunks

Ingredients:

- 1 cup low-fat cottage cheese
- 1 cup fresh pineapple chunks

Instructions:

1. Combine cottage cheese with pineapple chunks.
2. A quick and easy protein-packed snack.

Nutrition Information (per serving):

- Calories: 180
- Protein: 21g
- Carbohydrates: 22g
- Fat: 2g
- Fiber: 2g
- Sugar: 18g

- Portion Size: 1 cup cottage cheese with pineapple chunks

Mixed Nuts and Seeds Trail Mix

Ingredients:

- 1/4 cup almonds
- 1/4 cup walnuts
- 2 tbsp pumpkin seeds
- 2 tbsp sunflower seeds
- 1 tbsp dried cranberries

Instructions:

1. Combine almonds, walnuts, pumpkin seeds, sunflower seeds, and dried cranberries.
2. Portion into small servings for a crunchy, nutrient-rich snack.

Nutrition Information (per serving):

- Calories: 180
- Protein: 5g
- Carbohydrates: 10g
- Fat: 15g

- Fiber: 3g

- Sugar: 4g

- Portion Size: 1/4 cup mixed nuts and seeds trail mix

Edamame with Sea Salt

Ingredients:

- 1 cup edamame (frozen, thawed)
- Sea salt to taste

Instructions:

1. Steam or boil edamame according to package instructions.
2. Sprinkle with sea salt for a simple and protein-packed snack.

Nutrition Information (per serving):

- Calories: 120
- Protein: 11g
- Carbohydrates: 9g
- Fat: 5g
- Fiber: 4g
- Sugar: 2g

- Portion Size: 1 cup edamame with sea salt

Carrot and Celery Sticks with Greek Tzatziki

Ingredients:

- 2 carrots, cut into sticks
- 2 celery stalks, cut into sticks
- 1/2 cup Greek yogurt
- 1/4 cucumber, grated
- 1 clove garlic, minced
- 1 tbsp fresh dill, chopped
- Salt and pepper to taste

Instructions:

1. Arrange carrot and celery sticks on a plate.
2. In a bowl, mix Greek yogurt, grated cucumber, garlic, dill, salt, and pepper for the tzatziki dip.
3. Dip and enjoy this crunchy and flavorful combination.

Nutrition Information (per serving):

- Calories: 70
- Protein: 3g
- Carbohydrates: 12g
- Fat: 1g
- Fiber: 3g
- Sugar: 7g
- Portion Size: 1 cup mixed carrot and celery sticks with 1/4 cup tzatziki

Roasted Red Pepper and Feta Dip

Ingredients:

- 1 cup roasted red peppers (from a jar), drained
- 1/2 cup feta cheese, crumbled
- 2 tbsp olive oil
- 1 clove garlic, minced
- 1 tsp dried oregano
- Salt and pepper to taste
- Whole grain crackers for serving

Instructions:

1. In a food processor, blend roasted red peppers, feta cheese, olive oil, garlic, oregano, salt, and pepper until smooth.

2. Serve with whole grain crackers for a Mediterranean-inspired treat.

Nutrition Information (per serving):

- Calories: 120
- Protein: 4g
- Carbohydrates: 6g
- Fat: 9g
- Fiber: 2g
- Sugar: 3g
- Portion Size: 1/4 cup dip with 5 whole grain crackers

Avocado and Tomato Salsa

Ingredients:

- 2 avocados, diced
- 1 cup cherry tomatoes, quartered
- 1/4 cup red onion, finely chopped
- 1/4 cup fresh cilantro, chopped

- 1 lime, juiced
- Salt and pepper to taste
- Baked tortilla chips for serving

Instructions:

1. In a bowl, combine avocados, cherry tomatoes, red onion, cilantro, lime juice, salt, and pepper.
2. Serve with baked tortilla chips for a zesty and satisfying snack.

Nutrition Information (per serving):
- Calories: 160
- Protein: 2g
- Carbohydrates: 12g
- Fat: 13g
- Fiber: 7g
- Sugar: 2g
- Portion Size: 1/2 cup salsa with 10 baked tortilla chips

Hard-Boiled Eggs with Mustard

Ingredients:

- 2 hard-boiled eggs
- 1 tbsp mustard (Dijon or your preference)

Instructions:

1. Slice hard-boiled eggs in half.
2. Add a dollop of mustard on each egg half for a protein-packed and flavorful snack.

Nutrition Information (per serving):

- Calories: 140
- Protein: 12g
- Carbohydrates: 2g
- Fat: 9g
- Fiber: 0g
- Sugar: 0g
- Portion Size: 2 hard-boiled egg halves with mustard

Whole Grain Crackers with Cheese

Ingredients:

- 10 whole grain crackers
- 1 oz cheese (your choice), sliced

Instructions:

1. Arrange whole grain crackers on a plate.
2. Top each cracker with a slice of cheese for a satisfying and balanced snack.

Nutrition Information (per serving):

- Calories: 150
- Protein: 6g
- Carbohydrates: 15g
- Fat: 8g
- Fiber: 3g
- Sugar: 0g
- Portion Size: 10 whole grain crackers with 1 oz cheese

Mini Caprese Skewers

Ingredients:

- 14 cherry tomatoes
- 14 fresh mozzarella balls
- 14 fresh basil leaves
- Balsamic glaze for drizzling

Instructions:

1. Thread a cherry tomato, mozzarella ball, and basil leaf onto a small skewer.
2. Arrange skewers on a platter and drizzle with balsamic glaze for a classic and elegant snack.

Nutrition Information (per serving):

- Calories: 120
- Protein: 8g
- Carbohydrates: 5g
- Fat: 8g
- Fiber: 1g
- Sugar: 3g
- Portion Size: 7 mini caprese skewers

Smoked Salmon Cucumber Bites

Ingredients:

- 1 cucumber, sliced into rounds
- 4 oz smoked salmon
- 2 tbsp cream cheese
- Fresh dill for garnish

Instructions:

1. Spread a thin layer of cream cheese on each cucumber round.
2. Top with smoked salmon and garnish with fresh dill for an elegant and protein-rich bite.

Nutrition Information (per serving):

- Calories: 100
- Protein: 10g
- Carbohydrates: 2g
- Fat: 6g
- Fiber: 0g
- Sugar: 1g
- Portion Size: 5 smoked salmon cucumber bites

Chapter 6: Desserts

These treats are not only delicious but also designed to be mindful of your health, ensuring a sweet finale without compromising your well-being. Let's explore the art of creating desserts that tantalize your taste buds while keeping your blood sugar levels in check.

Sugar-Free Blueberry Muffins

Ingredients:

- 2 cups almond flour
- 1/2 cup coconut flour
- 1 teaspoon baking powder
- 1/2 teaspoon baking soda
- 1/4 teaspoon salt
- 1/2 cup unsweetened applesauce
- 1/4 cup almond milk
- 3 eggs
- 1 teaspoon vanilla extract
- 1 cup fresh blueberries

Instructions:

1. Preheat the oven to 350°F (175°C).

2. In a bowl, combine almond flour, coconut flour, baking powder, baking soda, and salt.

3. In another bowl, whisk together applesauce, almond milk, eggs, and vanilla extract.

4. Gradually add the wet ingredients to the dry ingredients, stirring until well combined.

5. Gently fold in the fresh blueberries.

6. Spoon the batter into muffin cups and bake for 20-25 minutes or until a toothpick comes out clean.

Nutrition Information (per serving):

- Calories: 150
- Protein: 6g
- Carbohydrates: 12g
- Fat: 9g
- Fiber: 3g
- Sugar: 2g
- Portion Size: 1 muffin

Dark Chocolate-Dipped Strawberries

Ingredients:

- 1 cup dark chocolate chips
- 1 tablespoon coconut oil
- Fresh strawberries, washed and dried

Instructions:

1. Melt dark chocolate chips with coconut oil in a heatproof bowl.
2. Dip each strawberry into the melted chocolate, ensuring even coating.
3. Place dipped strawberries on a parchment-lined tray.
4. Allow the chocolate to set in the refrigerator for at least 30 minutes.

Nutrition Information (per serving):

- Calories: 60
- Protein: 1g
- Carbohydrates: 7g
- Fat: 4g
- Fiber: 2g
- Sugar: 3g

- Portion Size: 3 strawberries

Baked Apples with Cinnamon

Ingredients:

- 4 medium-sized apples, cored and halved
- 1 tablespoon cinnamon
- 1 tablespoon melted coconut oil
- 2 tablespoons chopped walnuts (optional)

Instructions:

1. Preheat the oven to 375°F (190°C).
2. Place apple halves in a baking dish.
3. Drizzle melted coconut oil over the apples and sprinkle with cinnamon.
4. Bake for 25-30 minutes or until apples are tender.
5. Optionally, top with chopped walnuts before serving.

Nutrition Information (per serving):

- Calories: 120
- Protein: 1g
- Carbohydrates: 20g
- Fat: 5g

- Fiber: 4g

- Sugar: 15g

- Portion Size: 2 apple halves

Berry and Yogurt Popsicles

Ingredients:

- 1 cup mixed berries (strawberries, blueberries, raspberries)

- 1 cup plain Greek yogurt

- 1 tablespoon honey

- 1 teaspoon vanilla extract

Instructions:

1. Blend mixed berries, Greek yogurt, honey, and vanilla extract until smooth.

2. Pour the mixture into popsicle molds.

3. Insert popsicle sticks and freeze for at least 4 hours.

Nutrition Information (per serving):

- Calories: 70

- Protein: 5g

- Carbohydrates: 10g

- Fat: 1g
- Fiber: 2g
- Sugar: 7g
- Portion Size: 1 popsicle

Almond Flour Chocolate Chip Cookies

Ingredients:

- 2 cups almond flour
- 1/2 cup coconut oil, melted
- 1/3 cup sugar-free chocolate chips
- 1/4 cup almond butter
- 1/4 cup erythritol (or preferred sugar substitute)
- 1 teaspoon vanilla extract
- 1/2 teaspoon baking soda
- 1/4 teaspoon salt

Instructions:

1. Preheat the oven to 350°F (175°C).

2. In a bowl, mix almond flour, melted coconut oil, chocolate chips, almond butter, erythritol, vanilla extract, baking soda, and salt.

3. Form dough into cookies and place on a baking sheet.

4. Bake for 10-12 minutes or until edges are golden brown.

Nutrition Information (per serving):

- Calories: 120
- Protein: 3g
- Carbohydrates: 5g
- Fat: 10g
- Fiber: 2g
- Sugar: 1g
- Portion Size: 2 cookies

Greek Yogurt and Berry Parfait

Ingredients:

- 1 cup plain Greek yogurt
- 1/2 cup mixed berries (blueberries, strawberries)
- 1 tablespoon chia seeds
- 1 tablespoon honey

- 1/4 cup granola (sugar-free)

Instructions:

1. In a glass, layer Greek yogurt, mixed berries, chia seeds, and honey.
2. Repeat the layers until the glass is filled.
3. Top with granola before serving.

Nutrition Information (per serving):

- Calories: 180
- Protein: 15g
- Carbohydrates: 20g
- Fat: 5g
- Fiber: 4g
- Sugar: 12g
- Portion Size: 1 parfait

Avocado Chocolate Mousse

Ingredients:

- 2 ripe avocados
- 1/4 cup unsweetened cocoa powder
- 1/4 cup almond milk

- 1/4 cup maple syrup (or sugar substitute)
- 1 teaspoon vanilla extract
- Pinch of salt

Instructions:

1. Blend avocados, cocoa powder, almond milk, maple syrup, vanilla extract, and a pinch of salt until smooth.
2. Refrigerate for at least 1 hour before serving.

Nutrition Information (per serving):

- Calories: 150
- Protein: 3g
- Carbohydrates: 15g
- Fat: 10g
- Fiber: 7g
- Sugar: 6g
- Portion Size: 1/2 cup

Pumpkin Spice Chia Pudding

Ingredients:

- 1/4 cup chia seeds

- 1 cup unsweetened almond milk
- 1/4 cup pumpkin puree
- 1 tablespoon maple syrup (or sugar substitute)
- 1/2 teaspoon pumpkin spice

Instructions:

1. Mix chia seeds, almond milk, pumpkin puree, maple syrup, and pumpkin spice in a bowl.
2. Refrigerate overnight or until the mixture thickens.
3. Stir before serving.

Nutrition Information (per serving):

- Calories: 90
- Protein: 3g
- Carbohydrates: 11g
- Fat: 4g
- Fiber: 6g
- Sugar: 3g
- Portion Size: 1/2 cup

Coconut Flour Banana Bread

Ingredients:

- 1 cup coconut flour
- 1 teaspoon baking soda
- 1/4 teaspoon salt
- 3 ripe bananas, mashed
- 1/4 cup coconut oil, melted
- 1/4 cup almond milk
- 3 eggs
- 1 teaspoon vanilla extract

Instructions:

1. Preheat the oven to 350°F (175°C).
2. In a bowl, combine coconut flour, baking soda, and salt.
3. In another bowl, mix mashed bananas, melted coconut oil, almond milk, eggs, and vanilla extract.
4. Gradually add the wet ingredients to the dry ingredients, stirring until well combined.
5. Pour the batter into a greased loaf pan and bake for 45-50 minutes.

Nutrition Information (per serving):

- Calories: 120
- Protein: 4g
- Carbohydrates: 15g
- Fat: 6g
- Fiber: 7g
- Sugar: 5g
- Portion Size: 1 slice

Raspberry Sorbet

Ingredients:

- 2 cups frozen raspberries
- 1/4 cup fresh lemon juice
- 1/4 cup water
- 2 tablespoons honey (or sugar substitute)

Instructions:

1. Blend frozen raspberries, lemon juice, water, and honey until smooth.
2. Pour the mixture into a shallow dish and freeze for at least 4 hours.
3. Scoop and serve when ready.

Nutrition Information (per serving):

- Calories: 60
- Protein: 1g
- Carbohydrates: 15g
- Fat: 0g
- Fiber: 6g
- Sugar: 8g
- Portion Size: 1/2 cup

Nut and Seed Energy Balls

Ingredients:

- 1 cup mixed nuts (almonds, walnuts, cashews)
- 1/2 cup seeds (pumpkin seeds, sunflower seeds)
- 1/2 cup pitted dates
- 2 tablespoons chia seeds
- 1 tablespoon almond butter
- 1 teaspoon vanilla extract
- Pinch of salt

Instructions:

1. In a food processor, blend nuts, seeds, dates, chia seeds, almond butter, vanilla extract, and salt until a sticky dough forms.
2. Roll the mixture into bite-sized balls and refrigerate for at least 1 hour.

Nutrition Information (per serving):

*   Calories: 100
*   Protein: 3g
*   Carbohydrates: 8g
*   Fat: 7g
*   Fiber: 2g
*   Sugar: 5g
*   Portion Size: 2 balls

Lemon Poppy Seed Cake (Sugar-Free)

Ingredients:

*   1 cup almond flour
*   1/4 cup coconut flour

- 1/4 cup erythritol (or preferred sugar substitute)
- 1 teaspoon baking powder
- 1/4 teaspoon salt
- 1/4 cup melted coconut oil
- 1/4 cup lemon juice
- 2 tablespoons poppy seeds
- 3 eggs
- 1 teaspoon lemon zest

Instructions:

1. Preheat the oven to 350°F (175°C).
2. In a bowl, combine almond flour, coconut flour, erythritol, baking powder, and salt.
3. In another bowl, whisk together melted coconut oil, lemon juice, poppy seeds, eggs, and lemon zest.
4. Gradually add the wet ingredients to the dry ingredients, stirring until well combined.
5. Pour the batter into a greased cake pan and bake for 25-30 minutes.

Nutrition Information (per serving):

- Calories: 130

- Protein: 4g

- Carbohydrates: 7g

- Fat: 10g

- Fiber: 3g

- Sugar: 1g

- Portion Size: 1 slice

Vanilla Chia Seed Pudding with Fresh Mango

Ingredients:

- 1/4 cup chia seeds

- 1 cup unsweetened almond milk

- 1 tablespoon vanilla extract

- 1 tablespoon maple syrup (or sugar substitute)

- 1 ripe mango, diced

Instructions:

1. In a bowl, mix chia seeds, almond milk, vanilla extract, and maple syrup.

2. Refrigerate for at least 2 hours or overnight.

3. Top with fresh diced mango before serving.

Nutrition Information (per serving):

- Calories: 120
- Protein: 4g
- Carbohydrates: 18g
- Fat: 5g
- Fiber: 8g
- Sugar: 9g
- Portion Size: 1/2 cup

Strawberry Shortcake with Almond Flour Biscuits

Ingredients:

- 1 cup almond flour
- 1/4 cup coconut flour
- 1/4 cup erythritol (or preferred sugar substitute)
- 1 teaspoon baking powder
- 1/4 teaspoon salt
- 1/4 cup melted coconut oil
- 1/4 cup unsweetened almond milk
- 1 teaspoon vanilla extract
- Fresh strawberries, sliced

Instructions:

1. Preheat the oven to 350°F (175°C).

2. In a bowl, combine almond flour, coconut flour, erythritol, baking powder, and salt.

3. In another bowl, whisk together melted coconut oil, almond milk, and vanilla extract.

4. Gradually add the wet ingredients to the dry ingredients, stirring until well combined.

5. Drop spoonfuls of batter onto a baking sheet and bake for 15-18 minutes.

6. Allow the almond flour biscuits to cool, then assemble with sliced strawberries.

Nutrition Information (per serving):

- Calories: 150
- Protein: 4g
- Carbohydrates: 10g
- Fat: 11g
- Fiber: 3g
- Sugar: 5g
- Portion Size: 1 shortcake

Grilled Pineapple with Cinnamon

Ingredients:

- 1 pineapple, peeled, cored, and sliced
- 1 teaspoon coconut oil
- 1 teaspoon cinnamon

Instructions:

1. Preheat the grill or grill pan.
2. Brush pineapple slices with coconut oil.
3. Grill pineapple slices for 2-3 minutes on each side.
4. Sprinkle with cinnamon before serving.

Nutrition Information (per serving):

- Calories: 60
- Protein: 0g
- Carbohydrates: 15g
- Fat: 1g
- Fiber: 2g
- Sugar: 9g
- Portion Size: 1/2 cup

These delicious concoctions are not only a treat for your taste buds but also packed with essential nutrients to support your health. Whether you're craving a refreshing burst of tropical flavors or a comforting sip of chocolatey goodness, we've got you covered.

Green Detox Smoothie

Ingredients:

- 1 cup fresh spinach leaves
- 1/2 cucumber, peeled and sliced
- 1 green apple, cored and chopped
- 1/2 lemon, juiced
- 1 cup water or coconut water
- Ice cubes (optional)

Instructions:

1. Combine spinach, cucumber, green apple, and lemon juice in a blender.
2. Add water or coconut water for desired consistency.

3. Blend until smooth.

4. Add ice cubes if preferred.

5. Pour into a glass and enjoy!

Nutrition Information (per serving):

- Calories: 90

- Protein: 2g

- Carbohydrates: 22g

- Fat: 0.5g

- Fiber: 5g

- Sugar: 14g

- Portion Size: 1 serving

Berry Blast Smoothie

Ingredients:

- 1/2 cup strawberries, hulled

- 1/2 cup blueberries

- 1/2 cup raspberries

- 1/2 banana

- 1 cup unsweetened almond milk

- Ice cubes (optional)

Instructions:

1. Combine strawberries, blueberries, raspberries, banana, and almond milk in a blender.
2. Blend until smooth.
3. Add ice cubes if desired.
4. Pour into a glass and savor the berry goodness!

Nutrition Information (per serving):

- Calories: 120
- Protein: 3g
- Carbohydrates: 28g
- Fat: 2g
- Fiber: 8g
- Sugar: 15g
- Portion Size: 1 serving

Tropical Paradise Smoothie

Ingredients:

- 1/2 cup pineapple chunks
- 1/2 cup mango chunks
- 1/2 banana
- 1/2 cup coconut milk

- 1/2 cup water
- Ice cubes (optional)

Instructions:

1. Blend pineapple, mango, banana, coconut milk, and water until smooth.
2. Add ice cubes for a refreshing twist.
3. Pour into a glass, and transport yourself to a tropical paradise!

Nutrition Information (per serving):

- Calories: 150
- Protein: 2.5g
- Carbohydrates: 35g
- Fat: 5g
- Fiber: 4g
- Sugar: 22g
- Portion Size: 1 serving

Spinach and Banana Smoothie

Ingredients:

- 1 cup fresh spinach leaves

- 1 banana
- 1/2 cup plain Greek yogurt
- 1/2 cup almond milk
- 1 tablespoon chia seeds
- Ice cubes (optional)

Instructions:

1. Blend spinach, banana, Greek yogurt, almond milk, and chia seeds until smooth.
2. Add ice cubes if a cooler texture is desired.
3. Pour into a glass and enjoy this nutrient-packed green delight!

Nutrition Information (per serving):

- Calories: 130
- Protein: 7g
- Carbohydrates: 18g
- Fat: 5g
- Fiber: 5g
- Sugar: 8g
- Portion Size: 1 serving

Avocado and Kale Smoothie

Ingredients:

- 1/2 avocado, peeled and pitted
- 1 cup kale leaves, stems removed
- 1/2 cup cucumber, sliced
- 1/2 lime, juiced
- 1 cup coconut water
- Ice cubes (optional)

Instructions:

1. Combine avocado, kale, cucumber, lime juice, and coconut water in a blender.
2. Blend until smooth.
3. Add ice cubes for a chill factor.
4. Pour into a glass and relish the creamy goodness!

Nutrition Information (per serving):

- Calories: 140
- Protein: 4g
- Carbohydrates: 16g
- Fat: 8g
- Fiber: 7g

- Sugar: 5g

- Portion Size: 1 serving

Mango Tango Smoothie

Ingredients:

- 1 cup mango chunks

- 1/2 cup orange juice

- 1/2 cup Greek yogurt

- 1 tablespoon honey (optional)

- Ice cubes (optional)

Instructions:

1. Blend mango chunks, orange juice, Greek yogurt, and honey until smooth.

2. Add ice cubes for a refreshing twist.

3. Pour into a glass and dance to the mango tango!

Nutrition Information (per serving):

- Calories: 160

- Protein: 6g

- Carbohydrates: 32g

- Fat: 1g

- Fiber: 2g

- Sugar: 26g

- Portion Size: 1 serving

Blueberry Almond Butter Smoothie

Ingredients:

- 1/2 cup blueberries

- 1 tablespoon almond butter

- 1/2 banana

- 1 cup unsweetened almond milk

- 1 tablespoon flaxseeds

- Ice cubes (optional)

Instructions:

1. Blend blueberries, almond butter, banana, almond milk, and flaxseeds until smooth.

2. Include ice cubes if a cooler texture is desired.

3. Pour into a glass and relish the delightful combination of blueberries and almond butter!

Nutrition Information (per serving):

- Calories: 180

- Protein: 6g

- Carbohydrates: 22g

- Fat: 9g

- Fiber: 5g

- Sugar: 10g

- Portion Size: 1 serving

Cucumber and Mint Smoothie

Ingredients:

- 1/2 cucumber, peeled and sliced

- 1/2 cup fresh mint leaves

- 1/2 lime, juiced

- 1/2 cup coconut water

- 1/2 cup water

- Ice cubes (optional)

Instructions:

1. Blend cucumber, mint leaves, lime juice, coconut water, and water until smooth.

2. Add ice cubes for a refreshing kick.

3. Pour into a glass and savor the cool and invigorating taste!

Nutrition Information (per serving):

- Calories: 50
- Protein: 1g
- Carbohydrates: 12g
- Fat: 0.5g
- Fiber: 2g
- Sugar: 6g
- Portion Size: 1 serving

Protein-Packed Chocolate Smoothie

Ingredients:

- 1 scoop chocolate protein powder
- 1 tablespoon unsweetened cocoa powder
- 1/2 banana
- 1 cup almond milk
- 1 tablespoon almond butter
- Ice cubes (optional)

Instructions:

1. Blend chocolate protein powder, cocoa powder, banana, almond milk, and almond butter until smooth.

2. Add ice cubes for a thicker consistency.

3. Pour into a glass and indulge in this protein-rich chocolate delight!

Nutrition Information (per serving):

- Calories: 220
- Protein: 20g
- Carbohydrates: 18g
- Fat: 9g
- Fiber: 5g
- Sugar: 6g
- Portion Size: 1 serving

Pineapple Coconut Smoothie

Ingredients:

- 1/2 cup pineapple chunks
- 1/2 cup coconut milk
- 1/2 cup Greek yogurt
- 1 tablespoon chia seeds
- Ice cubes (optional)

Instructions:

1. Blend pineapple chunks, coconut milk, Greek yogurt, and chia seeds until smooth.

2. Add ice cubes for a tropical chill.

3. Pour into a glass and transport yourself to a beachside paradise!

Nutrition Information (per serving):

- Calories: 180
- Protein: 6g
- Carbohydrates: 22g
- Fat: 8g
- Fiber: 4g
- Sugar: 16g
- Portion Size: 1 serving

Cherry Almond Smoothie

Ingredients:

- 1/2 cup cherries, pitted
- 1/2 cup almond milk
- 1/2 cup plain Greek yogurt
- 1 tablespoon almond butter

- 1 tablespoon honey (optional)
- Ice cubes (optional)

Instructions:

1. Blend cherries, almond milk, Greek yogurt, almond butter, and honey until smooth.
2. Include ice cubes for a refreshing twist.
3. Pour into a glass and enjoy the delightful combination of cherries and almonds!

Nutrition Information (per serving):

- Calories: 160
- Protein: 7g
- Carbohydrates: 20g
- Fat: 6g
- Fiber: 3g
- Sugar: 15g
- Portion Size: 1 serving

Carrot Cake Smoothie

Ingredients:

- 1/2 cup carrots, peeled and chopped

- 1/2 banana
- 1/4 cup walnuts
- 1/2 teaspoon cinnamon
- 1 cup almond milk
- Ice cubes (optional)

Instructions:

1. Blend carrots, banana, walnuts, cinnamon, and almond milk until smooth.
2. Add ice cubes for a cooler texture.
3. Pour into a glass and relish the taste of carrot cake in liquid form!

Nutrition Information (per serving):

- Calories: 190
- Protein: 5g
- Carbohydrates: 18g
- Fat: 12g
- Fiber: 4g
- Sugar: 9g
- Portion Size: 1 serving

Peanut Butter Banana Smoothie

Ingredients:

- 1/2 banana
- 2 tablespoons peanut butter
- 1 cup almond milk
- 1/2 cup plain Greek yogurt
- 1 tablespoon honey (optional)
- Ice cubes (optional)

Instructions:

1. Blend banana, peanut butter, almond milk, Greek yogurt, and honey until smooth.
2. Add ice cubes for a frosty texture.
3. Pour into a glass and savor the classic combination of peanut butter and banana!

Nutrition Information (per serving):

- Calories: 250
- Protein: 10g
- Carbohydrates: 23g
- Fat: 15g
- Fiber: 3g

- Sugar: 14g
- Portion Size: 1 serving

Watermelon Mint Cooler

Ingredients:

- 1 cup watermelon, diced
- 1/2 lime, juiced
- 1 tablespoon fresh mint leaves
- 1/2 cup coconut water
- Ice cubes (optional)

Instructions:

1. Blend watermelon, lime juice, mint leaves, and coconut water until smooth.
2. Include ice cubes for a refreshing experience.
3. Pour into a glass and enjoy this hydrating watermelon mint cooler!

Nutrition Information (per serving):

- Calories: 60
- Protein: 1g
- Carbohydrates: 15g

- Fat: 0.5g
- Fiber: 1g
- Sugar: 11g
- Portion Size: 1 serving

Mixed Berry Protein Smoothie

Ingredients:

- 1/2 cup mixed berries (strawberries, blueberries, raspberries)
- 1 scoop vanilla protein powder
- 1/2 cup almond milk
- 1/2 cup Greek yogurt
- 1 tablespoon flaxseeds
- Ice cubes (optional)

Instructions:

1. Blend mixed berries, vanilla protein powder, almond milk, Greek yogurt, and flaxseeds until smooth.
2. Add ice cubes for a colder texture.
3. Pour into a glass and relish this protein-packed mixed berry delight!

Nutrition Information (per serving):

- Calories: 200
- Protein: 18g
- Carbohydrates: 22g
- Fat: 5g
- Fiber: 6g
- Sugar: 12g
- Portion Size: 1 serving

CONCLUSION

In concluding the "Type 2 Diabetes Cookbook for Seniors," we embark on a journey that extends beyond the realm of recipes and meal plans, reaching into the heart of a lifestyle dedicated to health and well-being. This comprehensive guide has been crafted with the utmost care and consideration for the unique dietary needs of seniors managing type 2 diabetes.

As we close the pages of this cookbook, it's essential to reflect on the profound impact that conscious eating can have on one's life. Beyond the delicious recipes that grace these chapters, we've laid the foundation for a sustainable approach to nutrition. The 30-day meal plan serves as a roadmap, offering not just a collection of recipes, but a holistic strategy for achieving and maintaining optimal health.

The breakfasts, lunches, dinners, snacks, desserts, and smoothies are more than culinary creations; they are gateways to a life of flavor, nourishment, and balance. From the vibrant colors of nutrient-rich vegetables to the lean proteins and whole grains that form the core of these recipes, each dish is a celebration of wholesome ingredients working harmoniously together.

But this book is not just about what you eat—it's about embracing a lifestyle that nurtures the body and soul. It's about making informed choices that empower seniors on their journey to managing diabetes with grace and resilience. The carefully curated recipes not only cater to taste buds but also prioritize blood sugar management, demonstrating that mindful eating can be both pleasurable and healthful.

As we bid farewell, let the lessons learned within these pages linger. May this cookbook serve as a constant companion, guiding seniors towards a path of sustainable health, mindful choices, and a future filled with vitality. Remember, the kitchen is not just a place to prepare meals; it's a space for transformation, healing, and joy. Here's to a vibrant, delicious, and healthful journey ahead—bon appétit and cheers to a life well-lived!